YOUR KNOWLEDGE HAS VALUE

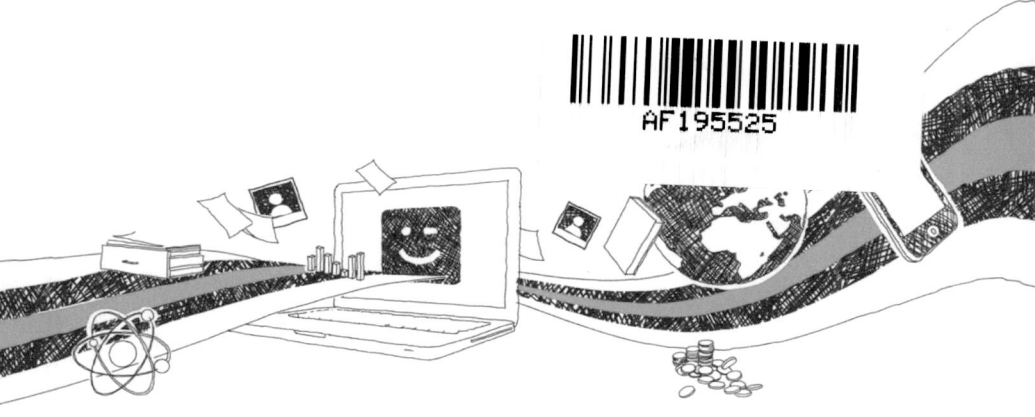

- We will publish your bachelor's and master's thesis, essays and papers

- Your own eBook and book - sold worldwide in all relevant shops

- Earn money with each sale

Upload your text at www.GRIN.com
and publish for free

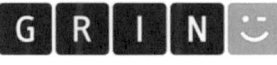

Bibliographic information published by the German National Library:

The German National Library lists this publication in the National Bibliography; detailed bibliographic data are available on the Internet at http://dnb.dnb.de .

This book is copyright material and must not be copied, reproduced, transferred, distributed, leased, licensed or publicly performed or used in any way except as specifically permitted in writing by the publishers, as allowed under the terms and conditions under which it was purchased or as strictly permitted by applicable copyright law. Any unauthorized distribution or use of this text may be a direct infringement of the author s and publisher s rights and those responsible may be liable in law accordingly.

Imprint:

Copyright © 2018 GRIN Verlag, Open Publishing GmbH
Print and binding: Books on Demand GmbH, Norderstedt Germany
ISBN: 9783668624719

This book at GRIN:

https://www.grin.com/document/388515

Patrick Kimuyu

Should Teenagers Be Given Access to Safe Medical Abortion In Order To Allow Them Complete Their Studies?

GRIN - Your knowledge has value

Since its foundation in 1998, GRIN has specialized in publishing academic texts by students, college teachers and other academics as e-book and printed book. The website www.grin.com is an ideal platform for presenting term papers, final papers, scientific essays, dissertations and specialist books.

Visit us on the internet:

http://www.grin.com/

http://www.facebook.com/grincom

http://www.twitter.com/grin_com

Should Teenagers Be Given Access to Safe Medical Abortion In Order To Allow Them Complete Their Studies?

Name: Patrick Kimuyu

Introduction 2

Arguments for Teen Abortion 2
    A Second Chance in School 2
    Reduce Teen Deaths 3
    Affirmative Approach 3
    Teenage Parenting Hinders Academic Excellence 4

Counter Arguments 4
    Psychological and Physical Risks 5
    Rebuttal 5

Conclusion 5

Works Cited 6

Introduction

Education is essential for a prosperous future for young people. This is why the United States educational system is designed to ensure that learners acquire the most valuable professional skills for career excellence. Over the years, reforms in the US educational system have always focused on improving intellectual competence of students. Despite the endless efforts by the US government, teachers and all stakeholders in the education sector, some challenges have always persisted; thus disrupting the learning process. This interferes with the smooth transitions from one level of education to the other and even college-to-work transition. One of the most challenging issues that have been disrupting the learning process in the US education system is teenage pregnancies. It is reported that about 750,000 cases of teenage pregnancies occur each year in the United States (Shuger 1). Of this population, two-thirds the affected teenagers are aged 18 and 19 years. As a result, over 200,000 abortion cases among teenagers are reported annually. However, teenage abortions occur at different rates across the US states. For instance, it is reported that over half of teenage pregnancies in New York, Minnesota, Mississippi, and New Jersey ends in abortion (Males 117). This implies that the desire to pursue academics contributes to the increase of abortion among teenagers. In light of these statistics, it is logical to allow teenagers to have safe medical abortion so as to pursue their academic dreams to prosperity. Therefore, this research paper will provide a logical discussion why teenagers should be allowed to access safe medical abortion.

Arguments for Teen Abortion

Currently, teenage abortion is legal in all 50 states in the United States. However, most state abortion laws require parental consent or evidence of judicial intervention. Therefore, it is worth noting that abortion among teenagers, as well as in all women is a legitimate practice under federal and states' law. However, most teenagers do not access safe medical abortion due to various reasons and this puts them at risk. From a logical perspective, allowing pregnant teenagers to access safe medical abortion has many beneficial implications in their education.

A Second Chance in School

Foremost, granting access to pregnant teenagers will enable teens to have a second chance to pursue their academic dreams. In most cases, teenage pregnancies disrupt education for the affected teens leading to school dropout. According to the National Conference of

State Legislatures (NCSL), only less than 2 percent of teenage mothers complete their education; whereas those who finish high school account for only 40 percent of teenage mothers (NCSL par. 2). This implies that the affected teens end up missing the basic educational skills to succeed in their careers. As such, they fall into the NEET (not on education, employment or training) which is characterized with failed transitions from adolescence to adulthood. Young people who are not in any training, education or education are known to experience enormous challenges in achieving socioeconomic sustainability. As a result, most of them develop antisocial behaviors. Therefore, teenage mothers are likely to experience similar consequences. In contrast, teenagers who pursue education to completion gain access to rewarding careers; thus enabling them to experience successful transitions into adulthood. As such, it is apparent that allowing teens to access safe medical abortion will grant them a second chance to continue their education to completion without having to drop out of school due to teenage pregnancies. This is so because school dropouts are related to teenage pregnancies (Shuger 1).

*Reduce Teen **Deaths***

The second reason why teens should be allowed access to safe medical abortion is that, it will reduce teen deaths related to unsafe abortions. In most cases, teenagers do not seek for abortion from medical facilities by their own because they are not informed of the right decisions to make. As a result, some of them seek assistance from their peers or unauthorized individuals to carry out abortion. This puts the lives of the affected teens at risk. One of the consequences which such teens face is death during or after abortion. On the other hand, some teens fail to obtain consent from their parents due fear because they do not want their parents to known that they are engaging in sexual behaviors. In such circumstances, teens rely on guidance from their peers which direct them towards unsafe methods of abortion. In the event of death owing to the consequences of unsafe abortion, both the education and lives of the concerned teens ends abruptly; thus, leading to a decrease in graduation rates. Therefore, allowing access to abortion for teens will reduce teen deaths during their academic lives.

*Affirmative **Approach***

From an educational perspective, gender inequalities in the US educational system have been found to have a negative impact on educational sustainability. This has prompted the government, as well as educators have been introducing affirmative initiatives to promote girl-child education.

Ordinarily, teenage girls experience the consequences of teenage pregnancies. In contrast, boys do not succumb to the adverse consequences of these pregnancies yet most of them are the key culprits. This phenomenon places the girl child in the disadvantaged group; thus affirmative approaches play significant roles in bridging the gender gap in the US educational system (Husain 1). Despite the impact of affirmative initiatives introduced in the US educational system, the tendency of dropping out of school by pregnant teens seems to hinder increased graduation of the girl-child. Therefore, creating awareness on safe medical abortion among teens will ensure that female teens remain in school and boost gender balance in education.

Teenage Parenting Hinders Academic Excellence

Moreover, teenage pregnancies have been found to cause psychosocial consequences to teenage mothers. Ordinarily, teenagers who give birth during their educational years face difficulties in pursuing their academics to completion. This is so because, parenting responsibilities deny them an opportunity to concentrate in their studies. Teenage pregnancies create faults in the cognitive development of teenage mothers owing to pressures of adulthood arising from failed transitions into adulthood (Manis 361). As a result, most teenage mothers show reduced performance in their learning.

Therefore, teenage pregnancies contribute to their failure in academics; the probable reason why a high percentage of teenage mothers complete their education. The consequence for poor academic performance among teenage mothers is failed college-to-work transition. In the current US labor market, professional competence which is evaluated by academic performance determines one's possibilities of accessing employment opportunities. Therefore, consequences of teenage pregnancies on those who struggle to college level compromise their employability.

Counter Arguments

Notwithstanding the benefits associated with teen abortions, especially educational benefits, some authors, as well, as professional experts claim that this practice bears negative impacts.

Psychological and Physical Risks

Some opponents observe that teen abortion exposes teens to psychological risks. For instance, Sobie and Reardon argue that teens who carry out abortion experience increased suicide tendencies. They also claim that these teenagers are more prone to psychological problems than adult women. In addition, they argue that most teens who abort experience troubled relationships (Sobie and Reardon par 3). On the other hand, Schulz and his colleagues argue that teenage abortion might cause cervical lacerations, physical injury to the mother's reproductive system (Schulz et al 1182).

Rebuttal

In rebuttal, the claim of psychological and physical risk is not adequate to justify opposition against allowing teenagers access to medical abortion. Foremost, these issues can be addressed through peer counseling programs which exist within the US educational system to ensure educational equity and justice (Thompson 310). Through peer counseling, post-abortion psychological effects can be countered; thus enabling survivors to experience remarkable cognitive development. On the other hand, physical risks can be minimized through safe abortion awareness campaigns. These awareness initiatives can be integrated into the existing gender-based affirmative campaigns.

Conclusion

In a brief conclusion, it is apparent that girl education in the United States, as well as the whole world, encompasses enormous challenges which have widened the gender gap. As a result, measures that aim at promoting successful learning up-to college graduation play paramount roles in ensuring socioeconomic sustainability of young people. Therefore, allowing teen's access to safe medical abortion appears to be one the most reliable approaches which promote girl-child education. This approach will provide teens with a second chance to pursue their studies to successful completion, as well as serving as an affirmative approach for bridging the current gender gap within the US educational system. However, this approach faces opposition from some experts which argue that it might increase psychological and physical risks among teenage abortion patients, but such outcomes can be addressed through counseling and awareness programs.

Works Cited

Husain, Muna. *Essays on Gender Differences in Education*. ProQuest, 2008. Print.

Males, Mike. *Teenage sex and pregnancy: modern myths, unsexy realities*. ABC-CLIO, 2010. Print.

Manis, Andrew. *Macon Black and White: An Unutterable Separation in the American Century*. Mercer University Press, 2004. Print.

National Conference of State Legislatures. *Postcard: teen pregnancy affects graduation rates*. Web. 6 Jan. 2018. < http://www.ncsl.org/research/health/teen-pregnancy-affects-graduation-rates-postcard.aspx>

Schulz, Kennedy et. al. "Measures to Prevent Cervical Injury During Suction Curettage Abortion." *The Lancet*, 1182-1184, 1993.

Shuger, Lisa. *Teen Pregnancy and High School Dropout: What Communities are Doing to Address These Issues*. Washington, DC: The National Campaign to Prevent Teen and Unplanned Pregnancy and America's Promise Alliance, 2012.

Sobie, Amy and Reardon David. "*Detrimental effects of adolescent abortion*." HTML File. Web. 7 Jan. 2018. < http://afterabortion.org/2001/detrimental-effects-of-adolescent-abortion/>

Thompson, Rosemary. *Professional school counseling: best practices for working in the schools*. Routledge, 2012. Print.

YOUR KNOWLEDGE HAS VALUE

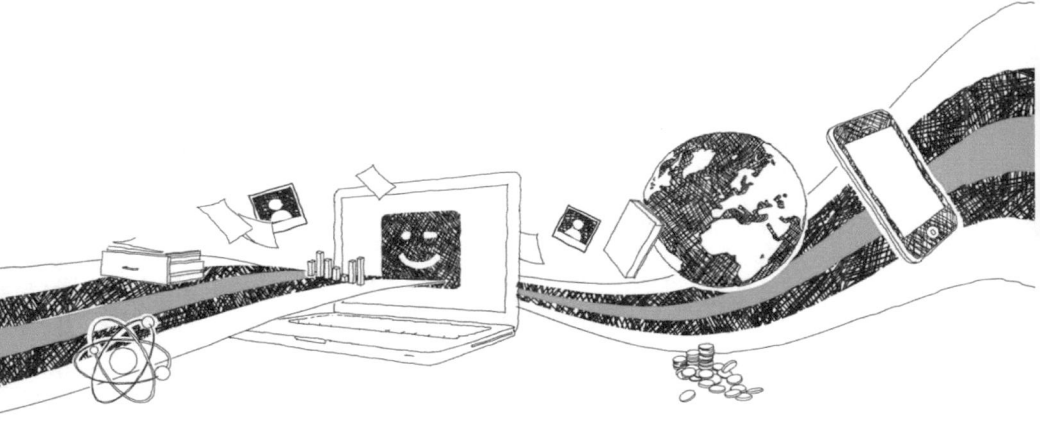

- We will publish your bachelor's and master's thesis, essays and papers

- Your own eBook and book - sold worldwide in all relevant shops

- Earn money with each sale

Upload your text at www.GRIN.com
and publish for free

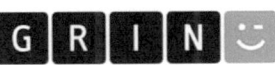